D.W. LINDSEY

Because We Care!

Caring for Aging Loved Ones: A Guide to Homecare for the Elderly

Table Of Contents

Chapter 1: Understanding the Aging Process

The Impact of Aging on Daily Activities

As our loved ones age, their ability to perform daily activities may be significantly affected. This subchapter explores the various ways in which aging can impact the daily activities of the elderly and offers insights and strategies to address these challenges. Targeted at caregivers, nurses, baby boomers, and grown children, this chapter aims to provide valuable information and guidance for those involved in homecare for the elderly.

One of the most common issues faced by the elderly is a decline in physical abilities. Simple tasks like getting dressed, bathing, or even walking may become increasingly difficult. In-home physical therapy can be a great solution to help maintain or regain mobility and independence. This subchapter delves into the benefits of in-home physical therapy and provides tips on finding the right therapists and exercises to improve strength and flexibility.

Another crucial aspect of aging that greatly impacts daily activities is cognitive decline. Dementia and Alzheimer's disease are prevalent among the elderly, leading to memory loss, confusion, and behavioral changes. Understanding the unique needs of individuals with dementia is essential for caregivers. Strategies for dementia care, including communication techniques and creating a safe environment, are discussed in this section.

Furthermore, home modifications can greatly enhance the safety and functionality of the living space for the elderly. From installing grab bars in the bathroom to ensuring proper lighting throughout the house, this subchapter provides practical advice on making necessary adjustments to accommodate the changing needs of aging loved ones.

Meal preparation and nutrition play a vital role in maintaining the health and well-being of the elderly. This chapter highlights the importance of proper nutrition for aging individuals and offers tips on meal planning, shopping, and preparing nutritious meals to address their specific dietary needs.

Medication management is another critical aspect of caregiving for the elderly. The chapter emphasizes the significance of understanding medication schedules, potential interactions, and side effects. It also provides guidance on organizing medications and developing effective systems for medication management.

Lastly, fall prevention and safety services are addressed in this subchapter. Falls are a leading cause of injury and hospitalization among the elderly. Caregivers and family members will find valuable insights on identifying potential hazards, implementing safety measures, and ensuring a safe environment to prevent falls.

In conclusion, this subchapter delves into the impact of aging on daily activities and provides a comprehensive guide for caregivers, nurses, baby boomers, and grown children involved in homecare for the elderly. Covering topics such as in-home physical therapy, dementia care, home modifications, meal preparation, medication management, and fall prevention, this chapter equips readers with the knowledge and strategies they need to provide effective care and support to their aging loved ones.

Common Health Concerns in Aging

As our loved ones age, it is important to understand the common health concerns that they may face. In this subchapter, we will discuss some of the most prevalent health issues that caregivers, nurses, baby boomers, and grown children should be aware of when caring for aging loved ones. By understanding these concerns, we can provide the best possible care and support for our elderly family members.

One of the most common health concerns in aging is dementia. Dementia affects millions of seniors worldwide and can have a profound impact on their daily lives. It is important to recognize the signs of dementia and seek early intervention and appropriate care. In this section, we will explore strategies and resources for providing dementia care for the elderly.

Another health concern that many aging individuals face is the need for physical therapy. As our loved ones age, they may develop mobility issues or experience a decline in their physical abilities. In-home physical therapy can be a great option to help improve strength, balance, and overall mobility. We will discuss the benefits of in-home physical therapy and provide tips for finding a qualified therapist.

Alzheimer's disease is another common health concern in aging. This progressive brain disorder affects memory, thinking, and behavior and can be challenging for both the individual and their caregivers. We will provide information on Alzheimer's care for the elderly, including strategies for managing symptoms and improving quality of life.

Home modifications are essential for ensuring the safety and comfort of aging loved ones. We will discuss the importance of home modifications for the elderly, such as installing grab bars, ramps, and stairlifts. These modifications can prevent falls and accidents and promote independence and mobility.

Nutrition is crucial for maintaining good health in aging individuals. We will explore meal preparation and nutrition services for the elderly, including tips for creating healthy and balanced meals. Additionally, medication management services for the elderly will be addressed, as many seniors require assistance with organizing and administering their medications.

Finally, fall prevention and safety services are vital for maintaining the well-being of aging individuals. Falls are a leading cause of injury among seniors, so it is essential to implement fall prevention strategies in the home. We will provide practical tips and resources for creating a safe environment and reducing the risk of falls.

By addressing these common health concerns in aging, caregivers, nurses, baby boomers, and grown children can ensure that their loved ones receive the best possible care and support. It is crucial to stay informed and seek appropriate resources and assistance to provide the highest quality of care for our aging loved ones.

Emotional and Psychological Changes in Aging

As our loved ones age, it is crucial for caregivers, nurses, baby boomers, and grown children to understand the emotional and psychological changes that occur. This knowledge is invaluable in providing effective care and support for elderly individuals. In this subchapter, we will delve into the various aspects of emotional and psychological changes that may arise with aging, and how to address them in the context of homecare for the elderly.

One of the most common emotional changes that occur in aging individuals is an increased susceptibility to depression and anxiety. Loss of independence, physical limitations, and the passing of friends and loved ones can all contribute to these feelings. Caregivers need to be aware of the signs of depression and anxiety, such as persistent sadness, loss of interest in activities, changes in appetite, and excessive worry. By recognizing these symptoms, caregivers can seek appropriate professional help and provide emotional support to their aging loved ones.

Another significant psychological change that may arise is cognitive decline, particularly in cases of dementia or Alzheimer's disease. Memory loss, confusion, and personality changes can be devastating for both the individual and their caregivers. It is crucial to educate caregivers on techniques for managing these conditions, such as creating a structured routine, providing visual cues, and engaging in memory-stimulating activities. Additionally, caregivers must take care of their mental well-being, seeking respite care when needed to prevent burnout.

In-home physical therapy is an essential aspect of caring for the elderly, especially those with mobility issues or chronic conditions. However, it is essential to recognize the emotional impact of physical limitations on the individual. Feelings of frustration, helplessness, and loss of self-esteem are common. Caregivers and physical therapists should approach these sessions with empathy, encouragement, and patience, helping the elderly individual maintain a positive mindset while achieving physical goals.

Lastly, caregiving can be physically and emotionally demanding, particularly when combined with other responsibilities. It is crucial for caregivers to prioritize self-care and seek support from others. Baby boomers and grown children who find themselves in the role of caregivers must acknowledge their own emotional needs and seek resources such as support groups, respite care, and counseling.

Understanding the emotional and psychological changes in aging is vital for providing holistic care to elderly individuals. By addressing these changes, caregivers, nurses, baby boomers, and grown children can create an environment that promotes emotional well-being, enhances quality of life, and fosters a loving and supportive relationship with their aging loved ones.

Chapter 2: Homecare for the Elderly

The Benefits of Homecare

Homecare for the elderly has become an increasingly popular and beneficial option for many families. In our fast-paced society, where individuals are busier than ever, providing care for aging loved ones can be a challenge. This subchapter aims to highlight the advantages of homecare for caregivers, nurses, baby boomers, and grown children who are looking for the best possible care for their elderly family members.

One of the most significant benefits of homecare is the comfort and familiarity it provides. Aging loved ones can remain in the comfort of their own homes, surrounded by their belongings and memories. This familiarity can have a positive impact on their mental and emotional well-being, reducing feelings of anxiety or confusion often associated with moving to an unfamiliar environment.

In-home care also promotes independence and allows elderly individuals to maintain their daily routines. Instead of conforming to the schedules of a facility, they can continue to engage in activities they enjoy, such as gardening, cooking, or even spending time with their pets. This sense of independence and control over their lives can significantly improve their overall quality of life.

Homecare services also offer specialized care for conditions such as dementia, Alzheimer's, and physical therapy needs. Trained professionals can provide personalized care plans tailored to the specific needs of each individual, ensuring they receive the appropriate level of support. This specialized care can help slow down the progression of certain conditions, enhance cognitive function, and improve physical mobility.

Furthermore, homecare services provide essential meal preparation and nutrition services, ensuring elderly individuals receive proper nourishment. Many aging adults struggle with maintaining a balanced diet, and having professionals who can assist with meal planning and preparation can greatly improve their health and well-being.

Medication management services are another vital aspect of homecare. Trained caregivers can help elderly individuals stay on top of their medication schedules, preventing any potential complications or missed doses. This level of support ensures their medications are taken correctly and can lead to better health outcomes.

Lastly, homecare services offer fall prevention and safety measures, reducing the risk of accidents and injuries. Caregivers can assess the home environment, making necessary modifications to enhance safety, such as installing grab bars, removing hazards, and ensuring proper lighting. These precautions provide peace of mind for both the elderly individual and their loved ones.

In conclusion, homecare for the elderly offers a wide range of benefits for caregivers, nurses, baby boomers, and grown children. From providing comfort and familiarity to specialized care and safety measures, homecare services can significantly improve the quality of life for aging loved ones. By choosing homecare, individuals can ensure their elderly family members receive the attention, support, and personalized care they need to thrive in their own homes.

Assessing the Needs of Aging Loved Ones

As caregivers, nurses, baby boomers, and grown children, it is essential to understand the unique needs of our aging loved ones. This subchapter aims to provide guidance on how to assess and address these needs effectively. Whether you are providing homecare for the elderly, specializing in dementia care, in-home physical therapy, Alzheimer's care, home modifications, meal preparation, medication management, or fall prevention and safety services, this information will prove invaluable.

When it comes to assessing the needs of aging loved ones, it is crucial to take a holistic approach. Firstly, consider the physical aspect. Observe any changes in mobility, balance, or strength. Are they experiencing difficulties with daily activities such as bathing, dressing, or walking? Are there any signs of chronic pain or health conditions that need attention? Identifying these issues will help determine the necessary support and care required.

Next, evaluate their cognitive function. Memory loss, confusion, and disorientation are common signs of dementia or Alzheimer's disease. Assess their ability to communicate, solve problems, and make decisions. Recognizing these cognitive changes will aid in tailoring appropriate care plans and interventions.

Additionally, assess their emotional and social well-being. Is your loved one experiencing loneliness, isolation, or depression? Evaluate their social interactions, interests, and hobbies. Understanding their emotional needs will allow you to incorporate activities that promote engagement, fulfillment, and mental well-being.

In assessing the needs of aging loved ones, it is essential to consider their living environment. Evaluate the safety and accessibility of their home. Are there any modifications required to prevent falls or accidents? Assess the need for assistive devices such as grab bars, ramps, or stairlifts. Ensuring a safe and comfortable living space is crucial for their overall well-being.

Lastly, don't overlook their dietary and medication needs. Assess their nutritional intake and any special dietary requirements. Evaluate their medication regimen and whether they require assistance with managing their prescriptions. Addressing these aspects will contribute to their physical health and overall quality of life.

By thoroughly assessing the needs of aging loved ones, caregivers, nurses, baby boomers, and grown children can provide the best possible care and support. Understanding the physical, cognitive, emotional, social, environmental, dietary, and medication needs will enable you to tailor homecare services accordingly. By addressing these needs holistically, you can ensure the well-being and happiness of your aging loved ones.

Creating a Safe and Comfortable Home Environment

As caregivers, nurses, baby boomers, and grown children, we understand the importance of providing a safe and comfortable home environment for our aging loved ones. This subchapter aims to guide you through the necessary steps to achieve just that. Whether you are caring for someone with dementia, Alzheimer's, or simply in need of general homecare for the elderly, these tips and strategies will help you create a space that promotes well-being and independence.

One crucial aspect of creating a safe home environment is assessing and modifying the physical surroundings. For those with mobility issues, in-home physical therapy can be a valuable resource. This service provides exercises and techniques to improve strength, balance, and coordination, minimizing the risk of falls. Additionally, considering home modifications such as grab bars, ramps, and handrails can enhance accessibility and ensure a safe living space for your loved ones.

In the case of dementia or Alzheimer's care, it is important to focus on eliminating potential hazards. This can be achieved by implementing safety measures such as installing locks on potentially dangerous areas, utilizing monitoring systems, and removing tripping hazards. Creating a calm and soothing atmosphere through proper lighting, familiar objects, and an organized living space can also help reduce anxiety and confusion.

Meal preparation and nutrition services play a vital role in maintaining the health and well-being of our aging loved ones. Ensuring a balanced diet that meets their nutritional needs is crucial. Collaborating with nutrition experts or meal delivery services can simplify this process, guaranteeing that your loved ones receive the necessary nutrients for their overall well-being.

Managing medications can be overwhelming, especially if multiple prescriptions are involved. Medication management services offer assistance in organizing medication schedules, refills, and potential interactions. This not only promotes safety but also provides peace of mind for both caregivers and their loved ones.

Finally, fall prevention and safety services are essential for maintaining a secure home environment. Identifying potential hazards, such as loose rugs or cluttered pathways, and implementing preventive measures such as installing handrails and adequate lighting can significantly reduce the risk of falls.

In conclusion, creating a safe and comfortable home environment is crucial for the well-being of our aging loved ones. By focusing on home modifications, dementia care, in-home physical therapy, meal preparation and nutrition services, medication management, and fall prevention, caregivers, nurses, baby boomers, and grown children can ensure the best possible care and quality of life for their elderly family members.

Chapter 3: Dementia Care for the Elderly

Understanding Dementia and its Types

Dementia is a progressive and debilitating condition that primarily affects older adults. As the number of seniors continues to rise, it is crucial for caregivers, nurses, baby boomers, and grown children to have a deep understanding of dementia and its various types. This subchapter aims to provide valuable insights into this complex disease, enabling individuals in the caregiving field to offer effective support and care to elderly loved ones suffering from dementia.

Dementia is not a specific disease but rather an umbrella term used to describe a range of symptoms that affect a person's memory, thinking, and social abilities. The most common form of dementia is Alzheimer's disease, accounting for approximately 60-80% of cases. Other types include vascular dementia, Lewy body dementia, frontotemporal dementia, and mixed dementia.

Alzheimer's disease, often characterized by memory loss and confusion, is caused by the accumulation of beta-amyloid plaques and tau tangles in the brain. Vascular dementia, on the other hand, is caused by reduced blood flow to the brain, leading to difficulties in thinking, reasoning, and memory. Lewy body dementia is associated with abnormal protein deposits in the brain, resulting in visual hallucinations, movement problems, and fluctuating alertness.

Frontotemporal dementia primarily affects the frontal and temporal lobes of the brain, leading to behavioral changes, language difficulties, and problems with decision-making. Mixed dementia refers to a combination of two or more types of dementia, often Alzheimer's disease and vascular dementia.

Understanding the specific type of dementia an individual is experiencing is crucial for providing appropriate care and support. Each type of dementia presents unique challenges and requires tailored interventions. Caregivers need to be well-versed in the symptoms, progression, and management strategies for each type of dementia to ensure the highest quality of care.

Moreover, this subchapter will explore the impact of dementia on the elderly, their families, and caregivers. It will discuss the emotional and psychological toll dementia can have on individuals, as well as the challenges faced by caregivers in managing the daily activities and behaviors of dementia patients.

By understanding dementia and its types, caregivers, nurses, baby boomers, and grown children can better anticipate the needs and provide compassionate care to their aging loved ones. This knowledge will empower them to make informed decisions about homecare, physical therapy, nutrition, medication management, fall prevention, and other essential services required to improve the lives of those living with dementia.

Communicating Effectively with Dementia Patients

When caring for aging loved ones with dementia, effective communication is crucial to maintaining their quality of life and overall well-being. Dementia can affect a person's ability to understand and express themselves, making it challenging for caregivers, nurses, and family members to connect with them on a meaningful level. In this subchapter, we will explore strategies and techniques for communicating effectively with dementia patients, equipping you with the tools you need to provide compassionate and person-centered care.

One of the key principles of communication with dementia patients is to use simple and clear language. Keep your sentences short and uncomplicated, using a calm and reassuring tone of voice. Avoid using complex or abstract concepts, as these may confuse or frustrate the individual. Instead, focus on using familiar words and phrases that they can easily grasp.

Non-verbal communication also plays a vital role in connecting with dementia patients. Maintain eye contact and use gentle touch to convey your presence and support. Facial expressions, gestures, and body language can help convey emotions and intentions when words fail. Be aware of your own non-verbal cues, ensuring they are warm, friendly, and non-threatening.

Listening actively is another essential aspect of effective communication. Give the person ample time to express themselves, even if their speech is slow or fragmented. Avoid interrupting or finishing their sentences, as this can be disempowering. Instead, show interest and empathy, responding with validation and understanding. Reflect their feelings and emotions, acknowledging their experiences without judgment.

Visual aids, such as photographs, can be powerful tools for communication. Displaying familiar pictures of family members, pets, or cherished memories can help trigger memories and facilitate conversation. Additionally, using written cues, such as signs or labels, can aid in navigation and reinforce routine tasks.

Finally, it is crucial to create a calm and supportive environment for effective communication. Minimize distractions, such as loud noises or excessive movement, which can increase agitation and confusion. Choose a quiet and comfortable space where you can engage in conversation without interruptions. Patience and flexibility are essential, as dementia patients may require extra time to process information and respond.

By implementing these strategies for effective communication, caregivers, nurses, and family members can foster meaningful connections with dementia patients. Remember, every individual is unique, and it may take time to find the best approach for each person. Nonetheless, by prioritizing empathy, patience, and understanding, you can make a positive difference in the lives of those living with dementia.

Providing Emotional Support for Dementia Patients

Dementia is a progressive condition that affects millions of elderly individuals worldwide. As caregivers, nurses, baby boomers, and grown children, it is crucial to understand the importance of providing emotional support to dementia patients. Emotional support plays a significant role in enhancing their quality of life and overall well-being.

Dementia can cause confusion, frustration, and anxiety in patients, making it challenging for them to communicate their needs effectively. By offering emotional support, caregivers can help alleviate these negative emotions and create a more positive and comforting environment.

One crucial aspect of emotional support is maintaining a calm and patient demeanor. Dementia patients often struggle with memory loss and may become easily frustrated or agitated. By remaining calm and patient, caregivers can help prevent escalated situations and provide a sense of security for the patient.

Active listening is another essential aspect of emotional support. Dementia patients may express themselves through nonverbal cues or fragmented speech. Caregivers should pay attention to these cues and respond with empathy and understanding. Engaging in meaningful conversations, even if they may not fully comprehend, can help dementia patients feel valued and connected.

Creating a familiar and nurturing environment is also crucial. Surrounding dementia patients with familiar objects, photographs, and music from their past can evoke positive memories and provide a sense of comfort. Engaging in activities that the patient enjoys, such as reading, puzzles, or listening to music, can stimulate their cognitive abilities and boost overall mood.

Additionally, it is important to involve family members and loved ones in the care process. Regular communication and updates on the patient's condition can help family members feel more connected and involved. Encouraging family visits and providing opportunities for them to engage with the patient can strengthen the support network and enhance the emotional well-being of the patient.

Lastly, self-care for caregivers is essential to be able to provide effective emotional support. Caring for a dementia patient can be emotionally draining and physically demanding. Taking breaks, seeking support from support groups or counseling services, and practicing self-care activities can help caregivers maintain their own emotional well-being and provide better support to the patients.

In conclusion, providing emotional support for dementia patients is vital for their overall well-being and quality of life. Caregivers, nurses, baby boomers, and grown children should understand the importance of remaining calm and patient, actively listening, creating a familiar environment, involving family members, and practicing self-care. By implementing these strategies, caregivers can make a significant positive impact on the lives of dementia patients, ensuring they feel loved, valued, and supported throughout their journey.

Chapter 4: In-Home Physical Therapy for the Elderly

The Importance of Physical Therapy for Aging Individuals

Physical therapy plays a crucial role in the overall well-being and quality of life for the elderly. As individuals age, they often experience a decline in physical abilities, which can lead to loss of independence and an increased risk of falls and injuries. However, with the help of physical therapy, these issues can be effectively addressed and managed.

One of the primary benefits of physical therapy for aging individuals is the improvement of mobility and balance. Through targeted exercises and techniques, physical therapists can help seniors regain strength, flexibility, and coordination. This, in turn, enables them to perform daily activities with greater ease and reduces the risk of falls, which is a common concern among the elderly.

In addition to improving physical function, physical therapy also aids in pain management. Many seniors suffer from chronic conditions such as arthritis, osteoporosis, or joint pain, which can greatly impact their quality of life. Physical therapists can develop personalized treatment plans that help alleviate pain and discomfort, allowing aging individuals to engage in activities they enjoy without limitations.

Furthermore, physical therapy can significantly contribute to the prevention and management of chronic diseases such as dementia, Alzheimer's, and cardiovascular conditions. Regular exercise and physical activity have been shown to enhance cognitive function, improve mood, and reduce the risk of memory decline. Physical therapists can design specialized programs that cater to the unique needs of individuals with these conditions, helping them maintain their cognitive abilities and overall well-being.

For caregivers, nurses, baby boomers, and grown children, understanding the importance of physical therapy for aging loved ones is crucial. By integrating physical therapy into their care plans, they can ensure that their elderly family members receive the necessary support to maintain their independence and enjoy an improved quality of life.

In conclusion, physical therapy is an essential component of caring for aging individuals. It enhances mobility, reduces pain, aids in the prevention and management of chronic diseases, and promotes overall well-being. By incorporating physical therapy into the care of aging loved ones, caregivers, nurses, baby boomers, and grown children can provide them with the highest level of care, allowing them to age gracefully and maintain their independence for as long as possible.

Assessing Mobility and Developing Personalized Exercise Plans

As caregivers, nurses, baby boomers, and grown children, we understand the importance of maintaining mobility and physical activity for the elderly. In this subchapter, we will delve into the topic of assessing mobility and developing personalized exercise plans to enhance the overall well-being of our aging loved ones.

When it comes to caring for the elderly, assessing their mobility is of utmost importance. Mobility issues can significantly impact their quality of life, leading to a decline in physical and mental health. By conducting a thorough mobility assessment, caregivers can identify any limitations or challenges their loved ones may have. This assessment entails evaluating their ability to walk, balance, climb stairs, and perform activities of daily living. Understanding their specific needs and limitations will allow caregivers to tailor exercise plans accordingly.

Developing personalized exercise plans is crucial for promoting optimal health and independence in the elderly. It is essential to consider their overall health condition, medical history, and any existing chronic conditions such as dementia, Alzheimer's disease, or physical impairments. By working closely with healthcare professionals, caregivers can design exercise plans that are safe, effective, and enjoyable for their aging loved ones.

In-home physical therapy services play a significant role in helping the elderly improve their mobility and overall fitness levels. These services focus on rehabilitation, strength training, and balance exercises, all of which can be tailored to individual needs. Incorporating physical therapy into an exercise plan can help prevent falls, enhance muscle strength, and improve overall mobility.

Additionally, home modifications are vital to ensure a safe environment for seniors. By making necessary adjustments such as installing grab bars, non-slip mats, and ramps, caregivers can reduce the risk of accidents and falls. A safe and accessible home environment is crucial for enabling seniors to engage in physical activity confidently.

Furthermore, meal preparation and nutrition play a pivotal role in maintaining overall health and wellness in the elderly. A well-balanced diet rich in nutrients can support muscle strength, bone health, and cognitive function. Caregivers should seek professional guidance to create personalized meal plans that meet the nutritional needs of their aging loved ones.

In conclusion, assessing mobility and developing personalized exercise plans are essential aspects of caring for aging loved ones. By conducting thorough mobility assessments, incorporating in-home physical therapy, making necessary home modifications, and focusing on proper nutrition, caregivers can enhance the overall well-being and quality of life of their elderly family members. It is crucial to collaborate with healthcare professionals to ensure the exercise plans are safe, effective, and tailored to individual needs.

Assisting with Daily Activities and Rehabilitation

When it comes to caring for aging loved ones, one of the most crucial aspects is providing assistance with their daily activities and rehabilitation. This subchapter aims to provide caregivers, nurses, baby boomers, and grown children with valuable insights into the necessary steps and strategies to ensure the well-being and quality of life for the elderly.

For individuals requiring homecare, it is essential to create a safe and comfortable environment that promotes independence and mobility. Home modifications play a vital role in achieving this goal. From installing grab bars in bathrooms to removing tripping hazards, these modifications can significantly reduce the risk of falls and accidents.

In-home physical therapy is another critical component of caring for the elderly. It offers a personalized approach to rehabilitation, allowing individuals to regain strength, improve mobility, and enhance overall well-being. This subchapter will provide guidance on how to find qualified physical therapists and the various exercises and techniques that can be implemented at home.

For those dealing with dementia or Alzheimer's, specialized care is necessary. Understanding the unique challenges and symptoms associated with these conditions is crucial for providing effective care. This subchapter will delve into the strategies and techniques that can help caregivers manage behavioral changes, promote cognitive stimulation, and create a supportive environment for their loved ones.

Meal preparation and nutrition services are also vital for the elderly. As individuals age, their nutritional needs change, and they may require assistance in planning and preparing healthy meals. This subchapter will explore meal planning options, discuss the importance of a balanced diet, and provide practical tips for ensuring proper nutrition.

Medication management is another crucial aspect of daily care. Keeping track of multiple medications, dosages, and schedules can be overwhelming. This subchapter will outline strategies for organizing medications, ensuring compliance, and seeking professional help when needed.

Lastly, fall prevention and safety services are essential for maintaining the well-being of the elderly. This subchapter will provide caregivers with valuable insights into identifying potential hazards, implementing safety measures, and creating a fall prevention plan tailored to the specific needs of their loved ones.

In conclusion, this subchapter on assisting with daily activities and rehabilitation in the book "Caring for Aging Loved Ones: A Guide to Homecare for the Elderly" offers valuable information and guidance for caregivers, nurses, baby boomers, and grown children. From home modifications to in-home physical therapy, dementia care, meal preparation and nutrition, medication management, and fall prevention, this subchapter covers a wide range of topics relevant to those caring for aging loved ones. By implementing the strategies and techniques outlined in this subchapter, caregivers can ensure the well-being and quality of life of their elderly family members or clients.

Chapter 5: Alzheimer's Care for the Elderly

Understanding Alzheimer's Disease and its Progression

Alzheimer's disease is a progressive neurological disorder that affects millions of people worldwide, especially the elderly population. As caregivers, nurses, baby boomers, and grown children, it is crucial to understand the nature of this disease and how it progresses to provide the best possible care for our aging loved ones.

Alzheimer's disease is characterized by the accumulation of abnormal proteins in the brain, leading to the formation of plaques and tangles. These plaques and tangles disrupt the communication between brain cells, causing memory loss, cognitive decline, and changes in behavior and personality.

The progression of Alzheimer's disease can be divided into three stages: early, middle, and late. In the early stage, individuals may experience mild memory lapses and difficulty finding the right words. They may also have trouble with problem-solving and organizing tasks.

During the middle stage of Alzheimer's, memory loss and confusion become more pronounced. Individuals may have difficulty recognizing family members and friends and may require assistance with daily activities such as dressing and bathing. Behavioral changes like agitation, aggression, and wandering may also occur.

In the late stage of Alzheimer's, individuals become completely dependent on others for their care. They may lose the ability to speak, walk, and perform basic tasks. Severe memory loss and cognitive decline make it challenging for them to recognize even their closest family members.

Understanding the progression of Alzheimer's is vital for caregivers, as it helps them anticipate the needs of their loved ones and provide appropriate care. It is crucial to establish a routine, maintain a safe and comfortable environment, and ensure proper nutrition and medication management.

Additionally, caregivers should consider home modifications to create a dementia-friendly space that minimizes accidents and promotes independence. Fall prevention and safety services are also essential to reduce the risk of injuries.

In-home physical therapy plays a crucial role in maintaining mobility and preventing muscle weakness and stiffness. Caregivers should work closely with therapists to develop a personalized exercise plan for their loved ones.

Furthermore, meal preparation and nutrition services are essential for ensuring that individuals with Alzheimer's receive a balanced diet. Adequate nutrition can help slow down the progression of the disease and improve overall health.

Medication management is another crucial aspect of Alzheimer's care. Caregivers should work closely with healthcare professionals to ensure that medications are taken as prescribed and to monitor any potential side effects.

In conclusion, understanding the progression of Alzheimer's disease is vital for caregivers, nurses, baby boomers, and grown children. By comprehending the different stages and their associated challenges, we can provide the best possible care for our aging loved ones. Implementing home modifications, in-home physical therapy, meal preparation and nutrition services, medication management, and fall prevention and safety services can greatly enhance the quality of life for individuals with Alzheimer's.

Creating a Structured Routine for Alzheimer's Patients

One of the most important aspects of caring for Alzheimer's patients is establishing a structured routine. Alzheimer's disease is a progressive brain disorder that affects memory, thinking, and behavior. Individuals with Alzheimer's often struggle with confusion and disorientation, and a structured routine can provide them with a sense of stability and familiarity.

Caregivers, nurses, baby boomers, and grown children play a vital role in the care of Alzheimer's patients. By following a structured routine, they can help manage the symptoms of the disease and improve the overall quality of life for their loved ones.

A structured routine involves establishing regular daily activities that are predictable and easy to follow. This routine should include activities that the individual with Alzheimer's is accustomed to and enjoys, such as meals, exercise, and social interaction. By incorporating these activities into their daily schedule, caregivers can help reduce anxiety and confusion.

When creating a structured routine for Alzheimer's patients, it is important to consider their individual needs and preferences. Some individuals may benefit from a more detailed schedule, while others may find a general outline of activities more helpful. Flexibility is key, as the needs of Alzheimer's patients may change over time.

In-home physical therapy can also be incorporated into the structured routine to help maintain physical function and mobility. By including exercises that promote strength and balance, caregivers can help prevent falls and promote overall well-being.

Meal preparation and nutrition services are essential for Alzheimer's patients. Caregivers should ensure that meals are prepared at regular intervals and that they include a balanced diet. This may involve adapting recipes to accommodate dietary restrictions or difficulty swallowing.

Medication management is crucial for individuals with Alzheimer's, as they may have difficulty remembering to take their medications on time. Caregivers should establish a medication schedule and ensure that medications are administered as prescribed.

Fall prevention and safety services should also be incorporated into the structured routine. Caregivers should make necessary home modifications to ensure a safe environment, such as installing grab bars in the bathroom or removing tripping hazards.

In conclusion, creating a structured routine is essential for Alzheimer's patients. By establishing a predictable daily schedule that includes meals, exercise, social interaction, medication management, and fall prevention measures, caregivers can provide a stable and supportive environment for their loved ones. This routine can help manage the symptoms of Alzheimer's and improve the overall well-being of the individual.

Managing Challenging Behaviors and Promoting Independence

As caregivers, nurses, baby boomers, or grown children, we are often faced with the task of caring for our aging loved ones. This responsibility comes with unique challenges, particularly when it comes to managing challenging behaviors and promoting independence in elderly individuals. In this subchapter, we will explore effective strategies and techniques that can be employed to address these issues, ensuring the well-being and quality of life for our elderly loved ones.

One of the most common challenges faced in caregiving is dealing with challenging behaviors, especially in individuals with dementia or Alzheimer's disease. These behaviors may include agitation, aggression, wandering, and resistance to care. To effectively manage these behaviors, it is important to understand the underlying causes. This can involve identifying triggers, such as fatigue, hunger, pain, or discomfort, and addressing them accordingly. Creating a calm and structured environment, establishing routines, and engaging in meaningful activities can also help reduce challenging behaviors.

Promoting independence is another crucial aspect of caregiving. While it is natural to want to assist our loved ones in every aspect of their daily lives, it is equally important to encourage their independence and autonomy. This can be achieved by allowing them to make choices whenever possible, involving them in decision-making processes, and providing opportunities for engagement and social interaction. Simple modifications to the home environment, such as grab bars, handrails, and adaptive equipment, can also facilitate independent living.

In addition to managing challenging behaviors and promoting independence, this subchapter also delves into other important topics related to homecare for the elderly. These include in-home physical therapy, meal preparation and nutrition services, medication management, fall prevention and safety services, and home modifications.

In-home physical therapy can greatly benefit elderly individuals by improving mobility, strength, and overall functioning. This section provides insights into the various exercises and techniques that can be incorporated into a physical therapy regimen.

Meal preparation and nutrition services play a vital role in maintaining the health and well-being of the elderly. Here, we discuss the importance of a well-balanced diet, provide tips for meal planning, and explore services that can assist in ensuring proper nutrition for our loved ones.

Medication management services are crucial for elderly individuals who may be taking multiple medications. This subchapter offers guidance on organizing medication schedules, understanding potential side effects, and ensuring adherence to prescribed regimens.

Fall prevention and safety services are essential to minimize the risk of accidents and injuries. We explore strategies for creating a safe living environment, including removing hazards, installing safety equipment, and promoting regular exercise.

Lastly, we address the topic of home modifications for the elderly. This section provides practical advice on adapting the home to accommodate the changing needs of our loved ones, such as installing ramps, widening doorways, and improving accessibility.

By understanding and implementing the strategies discussed in this subchapter, caregivers, nurses, baby boomers, and grown children can effectively manage challenging behaviors and promote independence in their aging loved ones. Additionally, they can access valuable information on other crucial aspects of homecare for the elderly, ensuring a safe, comfortable, and fulfilling environment for those in their care.

Chapter 6: Home Modifications for the Elderly

Identifying Home Safety Hazards

When it comes to caring for aging loved ones, one of the most important aspects is ensuring their safety at home. As caregivers, nurses, baby boomers, or grown children, it is crucial to be aware of the potential hazards that may exist in their living environment. This subchapter, "Identifying Home Safety Hazards," aims to provide you with essential information and practical tips to create a safe and secure home for elderly individuals.

One of the primary concerns when it comes to home safety is preventing falls. Falls can have devastating consequences for older adults, leading to fractures, head injuries, and a loss of independence. Therefore, it is crucial to identify and eliminate potential fall hazards. This section will guide you through a comprehensive home assessment, highlighting common hazards such as loose rugs, cluttered walkways, inadequate lighting, and unstable furniture.

Additionally, this subchapter will address the specific safety considerations for individuals with dementia or Alzheimer's. Cognitive impairments can make individuals more prone to accidents, wandering, or confusion. Understanding how to secure the home environment and implement appropriate measures to prevent accidents is vital for their well-being.

Furthermore, we will explore the importance of home modifications to accommodate the changing needs of the elderly. From installing grab bars in the bathroom to improving accessibility through ramps or stairlifts, making necessary adjustments to the home environment can significantly enhance their safety and independence.

In this chapter, we will also delve into the significance of proper medication management, meal preparation, and nutrition services for the elderly. These topics are essential components of homecare, as they directly impact their overall health and well-being.

Lastly, we will provide you with valuable insights into in-home physical therapy for the elderly. Physical therapy plays a crucial role in maintaining strength, balance, and mobility, thereby reducing the risk of falls and enhancing their quality of life.

By understanding and addressing the various safety hazards that may exist in a home, caregivers, nurses, baby boomers, and grown children can create a secure and nurturing environment for their aging loved ones. This subchapter aims to equip you with the knowledge and tools needed to ensure the well-being and safety of elderly individuals in their own homes.

Adapting the Home for Aging in Place

As our loved ones age, it becomes increasingly important to create a safe and comfortable environment for them to live in. Adapting the home for aging in place is a crucial step in ensuring their well-being and quality of life. In this subchapter, we will explore various modifications and services that can be implemented to meet the unique needs of our elderly family members.

One of the key considerations when adapting the home is to create a barrier-free living space. This involves removing tripping hazards such as loose carpets and ensuring that doorways are wide enough to accommodate mobility aids like wheelchairs or walkers. Installing grab bars in the bathroom and along stairways can provide additional support and prevent falls. Additionally, consider installing ramps to provide easy access to the home for those with limited mobility.

Another aspect to address is dementia care for the elderly. Creating a familiar and structured environment can greatly benefit individuals with dementia. Labeling drawers and cabinets, using color-coded signs, and providing clear visual cues can help them navigate their surroundings independently and reduce confusion. Installing safety locks on potentially hazardous areas, such as the kitchen or garage, can also prevent accidents.

In-home physical therapy is essential for maintaining the mobility and strength of aging individuals. By incorporating exercise equipment, such as resistance bands or small weights, into the home, seniors can engage in regular physical activity. It is also important to ensure that the home is designed with ample space for movement and that furniture is arranged to promote safety and accessibility.

Meal preparation and nutrition services play a vital role in the overall well-being of our elderly loved ones. Consider investing in meal delivery services that provide nutritious and balanced meals tailored to their dietary needs. Additionally, creating a well-equipped kitchen with easy-to-reach utensils and appliances can encourage them to prepare their own meals and maintain their independence.

Medication management services are crucial for seniors who require multiple medications. Implementing pill organizers and setting up reminders can help prevent missed doses or accidental overdoses. It is also advisable to keep a record of their medications and schedule regular medication reviews with healthcare professionals.

Lastly, fall prevention and safety services are paramount in protecting our aging family members. Installing adequate lighting throughout the home, removing clutter, and securing rugs and carpets can minimize the risk of falls. It is also advisable to conduct regular safety checks to identify potential hazards and address them promptly.

Adapting the home for aging in place is a multifaceted process that requires careful consideration of the specific needs of our elderly loved ones. By implementing these modifications and services, caregivers, nurses, baby boomers, and grown children can create a safe and comfortable environment that promotes independence, happiness, and overall well-being.

Assistive Devices and Technology for Independent Living

In today's fast-paced world, advancements in technology have made our lives easier and more convenient. This is no exception when it comes to caring for our aging loved ones. Assistive devices and technology have revolutionized the way we provide care and support to the elderly, allowing them to maintain independence and dignity in their own homes. In this subchapter, we will explore the various assistive devices and technologies available for independent living, catering to the specific needs of caregivers, nurses, baby boomers, and grown children.

When it comes to homecare for the elderly, assistive devices play a crucial role in enhancing their quality of life. From mobility aids such as walkers and wheelchairs to adaptive equipment like grab bars and raised toilet seats, these devices enable seniors to move around safely and comfortably within their homes. Additionally, technology has introduced smart home systems that can be programmed to control lighting, temperature, and security, promoting a sense of security and convenience.

For those caring for individuals with dementia or Alzheimer's, specialized technologies can provide peace of mind. GPS tracking devices, for instance, can be worn by dementia patients, enabling caregivers to locate them if they wander off. Medication management devices are also invaluable, ensuring timely and accurate administration of medications, reducing the risk of missed doses or overdose.

In-home physical therapy has become increasingly popular for the elderly, and technology has made it more accessible than ever. Virtual physical therapy sessions, conducted through video calls with certified therapists, allow seniors to receive expert guidance and exercises tailored to their specific needs from the comfort of their own homes. This not only saves time and effort but also encourages independence and active participation in their rehabilitation.

Home modifications are often necessary to create a safe and accessible environment for the elderly. From installing ramps and stair lifts to widening doorways and lowering countertops, these modifications enable seniors to navigate their homes with ease. Furthermore, assistive technologies such as fall detection devices and emergency response systems can provide immediate assistance in case of accidents or emergencies.

Nutrition and medication management are critical aspects of elderly care. Meal preparation services, delivered directly to their homes, ensure that seniors receive balanced and nutritious meals while adhering to any dietary restrictions. Medication management services, on the other hand, offer timely reminders and assistance with medication administration, reducing the risk of medication errors and improving overall health outcomes.

Fall prevention and safety services are paramount for the elderly, especially those with mobility issues. Assistive devices like bed rails, non-slip mats, and grab bars can significantly reduce the risk of falls, while safety technologies such as motion sensor lighting and home security systems enhance security and peace of mind.

As caregivers, nurses, baby boomers, and grown children, it is crucial to stay informed about the latest assistive devices and technologies available for independent living. By harnessing the power of technology, we can provide our aging loved ones with the support and care they need while preserving their autonomy and dignity.

Chapter 7: Meal Preparation and Nutrition Services for the Elderly

Assessing Nutritional Needs of Aging Loved Ones

Proper nutrition plays a crucial role in maintaining the health and well-being of our aging loved ones. As caregivers, nurses, baby boomers, and grown children, it is essential for us to understand the specific nutritional needs of the elderly, especially those suffering from dementia, Alzheimer's, or other age-related conditions. This subchapter will provide valuable insights on how to assess and meet the nutritional requirements of our aging loved ones, ensuring their overall health and quality of life.

When it comes to homecare for the elderly, it is vital to evaluate their nutritional needs regularly. As individuals age, their bodies undergo various changes that can impact their dietary requirements. Metabolism slows down, muscle mass decreases, and chronic conditions may develop, making it necessary to adjust their diet accordingly. By assessing their nutritional needs, we can identify any deficiencies or specific dietary restrictions and tailor their meals accordingly.

For those caring for elderly individuals with dementia or Alzheimer's, nutrition becomes even more critical. These conditions often lead to forgetfulness, confusion, and difficulty with eating and swallowing. It is crucial to ensure that meals are visually appealing, easy to eat, and nutritionally dense. Consulting with a nutritionist or dietitian who specializes in dementia care can provide valuable guidance in creating well-balanced and appropriate meal plans.

In-home physical therapy for the elderly is another niche that can greatly benefit from proper nutrition. Physical therapy aims to improve mobility, strength, and overall physical well-being. Adequate nutrition plays a significant role in supporting these goals. By assessing the nutritional needs of aging loved ones undergoing physical therapy, caregivers and therapists can develop meal plans that promote muscle growth, enhance bone health, and aid in the recovery process.

Furthermore, this subchapter will explore the importance of home modifications for the elderly in relation to nutrition. Creating a safe and accessible kitchen environment ensures that aging loved ones can easily prepare meals and maintain their independence. Simple modifications like installing grab bars, lowering countertops, or using non-slip flooring can significantly reduce the risk of accidents and falls while cooking.

Lastly, the subchapter will touch upon the significance of meal preparation and nutrition services, medication management, and fall prevention and safety services for the elderly. These services complement each other in providing well-rounded care for aging loved ones. By assessing their nutritional needs, caregivers can work with nutritionists, meal delivery services, and medical professionals to ensure that seniors are receiving proper nutrition, managing their medications effectively, and living in a safe environment that minimizes the risk of falls and accidents.

In conclusion, assessing the nutritional needs of our aging loved ones is a fundamental aspect of caregiving. By understanding their specific dietary requirements, we can provide the necessary support and ensure their overall health and well-being. Whether it is through proper meal planning, home modifications, or utilizing professional services, addressing the nutritional needs of the elderly enhances their quality of life and allows them to age gracefully.

Planning and Preparing Nutritious Meals

As caregivers, nurses, baby boomers, and grown children, we understand the importance of providing our aging loved ones with nutritious meals. Planning and preparing meals that meet their dietary needs can significantly contribute to their overall health and well-being. In this subchapter, we will discuss essential tips and strategies for planning and preparing nutritious meals for the elderly.

When it comes to meal planning, it is crucial to consider the dietary restrictions and preferences of our aging loved ones. Many elderly individuals may have specific health conditions that require dietary modifications. For example, those with diabetes may need to monitor their carbohydrate intake, while individuals with heart disease may need to limit their sodium intake. By understanding their unique needs, we can create meal plans that cater to their specific requirements.

To ensure our aging loved ones receive the necessary nutrients, it is essential to include a variety of food groups in their meals. A balanced meal should consist of lean proteins, such as fish, poultry, or legumes, along with whole grains, fruits, vegetables, and healthy fats. Incorporating a rainbow of colorful fruits and vegetables not only adds visual appeal but also provides a wide range of essential vitamins and minerals.

In addition to the content of the meal, the presentation and texture of the food can also impact the elderly's appetite. As we age, our taste buds and sense of smell diminish, making it vital to enhance the flavor of the food. Adding herbs, spices, and seasonings can make meals more enjoyable. Moreover, ensuring the food is visually appealing and has a variety of textures can help stimulate appetite. For example, incorporating crunchy vegetables or tender meats can make the dining experience more pleasurable.

Meal preparation should also take into account any physical limitations our aging loved ones may have. For individuals with limited dexterity or mobility, it may be necessary to prepare easy-to-eat finger foods or utilize specialized utensils that make self-feeding easier. Moreover, considering portion sizes and meal frequency can help maintain a healthy weight and prevent overeating or malnutrition.

In conclusion, planning and preparing nutritious meals for our aging loved ones is essential for their overall well-being. By understanding their dietary needs, incorporating a variety of food groups, enhancing flavors, and considering their physical limitations, we can ensure they receive the necessary nutrients. Providing them with delicious and visually appealing meals not only supports their health but also promotes a positive dining experience. Remember, every meal is an opportunity to show our love and care for our aging loved ones.

Addressing Dietary Restrictions and Medical Conditions

When caring for aging loved ones, it is important to consider any dietary restrictions or medical conditions they may have. This subchapter aims to provide caregivers, nurses, baby boomers, and grown children with valuable information on how to address these concerns effectively.

One of the most common dietary restrictions among the elderly is related to medical conditions such as diabetes, high blood pressure, or heart disease. It is crucial to work closely with healthcare professionals to develop a meal plan that meets their nutritional needs while managing their condition. This may involve reducing sodium, sugar, or fat intake and ensuring a balanced diet with plenty of fruits, vegetables, and lean proteins.

For individuals with dementia or Alzheimer's, mealtime can be particularly challenging. They may experience difficulties with swallowing, forget to eat, or have trouble recognizing food. In these cases, it is important to create a safe and calm environment, offering meals in small, manageable portions and using visually appealing plates and utensils. Additionally, caregivers should closely monitor their loved ones' food intake to ensure they are eating enough and receiving essential nutrients.

Homecare for the elderly may involve in-home physical therapy to maintain mobility and prevent further decline. Caregivers should collaborate with physical therapists to develop personalized exercise plans that accommodate any medical conditions or physical limitations. These plans may include stretching exercises, strength training, and balance exercises to reduce the risk of falls.

Medication management is another critical aspect of caring for aging loved ones. Caregivers should keep a detailed record of all medications, including dosages and schedules, to ensure they are administered correctly. It is essential to communicate with healthcare professionals regularly to review and update medication plans, as changes may occur over time.

Lastly, fall prevention and safety services are crucial for the elderly, as falls can lead to severe injuries. Caregivers should assess the home environment for potential hazards, such as loose rugs or poor lighting, and make necessary modifications. Installing handrails, grab bars, and non-slip mats can greatly reduce the risk of falls.

In conclusion, addressing dietary restrictions and medical conditions is an integral part of providing quality care for aging loved ones. By working closely with healthcare professionals, caregivers can develop personalized meal plans, manage medications effectively, and provide a safe environment to promote overall well-being.

Chapter 8: Medication Management Services for the Elderly

Understanding Medication Regimens and Potential Risks

As a caregiver, nurse, baby boomer, or grown child responsible for the care of an aging loved one, it is essential to have a comprehensive understanding of medication regimens and the potential risks associated with them. Medications play a critical role in managing various health conditions and improving the quality of life for elderly individuals. However, improper use or lack of knowledge about medications can result in adverse effects, drug interactions, and even hospitalizations. In this subchapter, we will explore the importance of understanding medication regimens and provide valuable insights into mitigating potential risks.

One of the first steps in managing medication regimens is to create a detailed list of all the medications your loved one is taking. This list should include the name of the medication, dosage, frequency, and any specific instructions provided by healthcare professionals. It is crucial to update this list regularly and share it with other healthcare providers involved in your loved one's care, including doctors, pharmacists, and nurses. This comprehensive medication list serves as a valuable reference and helps prevent medication errors, such as double-dosing or missing doses.

Understanding the potential risks associated with medications is equally important. Many medications have specific side effects that can impact an elderly individual differently than a younger person. For instance, certain medications may cause dizziness or drowsiness, increasing the risk of falls. It is crucial to be aware of these potential side effects and discuss them with healthcare providers. Additionally, being knowledgeable about potential drug interactions is vital, as some medications may interact adversely with others, leading to reduced effectiveness or increased side effects.

Regular communication with healthcare professionals is essential to ensure the safe and effective use of medications. Be proactive in asking questions, seeking clarification, and expressing concerns regarding your loved one's medication regimen. Pharmacists can be a valuable resource in providing medication education and checking for potential drug interactions. Additionally, healthcare providers can offer guidance on proper medication administration techniques and potential lifestyle modifications that may enhance the effectiveness of medications.

In conclusion, understanding medication regimens and potential risks is vital for caregivers, nurses, baby boomers, and grown children involved in the care of aging loved ones. By creating a comprehensive medication list, being aware of potential side effects and drug interactions, and maintaining open communication with healthcare professionals, you can ensure the safe and effective use of medications for your loved one. Taking these proactive steps will not only enhance their quality of life but also reduce the risk of medication-related complications.

Organizing Medications and Administering Dosages

As a caregiver, nurse, or family member responsible for the wellbeing of an aging loved one, one of the crucial tasks you may need to handle is managing their medications. Organizing medications and administering dosages correctly is essential to ensure their health and safety. In this subchapter, we will discuss effective strategies and tips to help you navigate this important aspect of homecare for the elderly.

First and foremost, it is essential to create a medication management system that works for you and your loved one. This system should include a clear schedule for when medications are to be taken and in what dosages. Depending on the complexity of the medication regimen, you may find it helpful to use pill organizers or digital medication management apps to keep track of the various medications and their corresponding dosages.

When organizing medications, it is crucial to keep them in a safe and easily accessible place. A locked cabinet or drawer can help prevent accidental ingestion or misuse, especially if there are children or others who may have access to the medication. Additionally, ensure that all medications are stored in their original containers, properly labeled with the name of the medication, dosage instructions, and expiration date.

Administering dosages correctly is equally important. Make sure you fully understand the instructions provided by the healthcare professional and follow them precisely. If there are any concerns or questions, do not hesitate to reach out to a pharmacist or healthcare provider for clarification.

In some cases, elderly individuals may have difficulty swallowing pills or may require assistance with self-administration. If this is the case, consider alternative medication forms, such as liquids or patches, which may be easier to swallow or apply. If assistance is needed, ensure you are trained in proper techniques, such as the use of pill splitters or crushing medications if appropriate.

Regularly reviewing and updating the medication regimen is essential, especially if multiple healthcare providers are involved. Keep an updated list of all medications, including over-the-counter drugs and supplements, and share it with the healthcare team to avoid any potential drug interactions or duplications.

Remember, organizing medications and administering dosages requires careful attention and organization. By implementing an effective medication management system and staying informed, you can ensure the wellbeing and safety of your aging loved one.

Collaboration with Healthcare Professionals for Medication Safety

One of the most critical aspects of caring for aging loved ones is ensuring their medication safety. Medications play a crucial role in managing various health conditions, but can also pose significant risks if not managed properly. As caregivers, nurses, baby boomers, and grown children, it is essential to collaborate with healthcare professionals to ensure the well-being of our elderly loved ones.

Healthcare professionals, including doctors, pharmacists, and nurses, possess specialized knowledge and expertise in medication management. By working closely with them, we can ensure that our aging loved ones receive the right medications, in the correct doses, and at the appropriate times. This collaboration can significantly reduce the risk of medication errors, adverse drug reactions, and potential hospitalizations.

To initiate collaboration, it is essential to establish open lines of communication with healthcare professionals involved in our loved one's care. This includes regular visits to primary care physicians, specialists, and pharmacists. During these visits, it is crucial to provide accurate and up-to-date information about the medications our loved ones are taking, including prescription drugs, over-the-counter medications, and any supplements. This information helps healthcare professionals make informed decisions regarding medication management.

Additionally, caregivers should actively participate in medication reviews and discussions. By asking questions and seeking clarification, we can gain a better understanding of the purpose, side effects, and potential interactions of the medications prescribed to our loved ones. This knowledge empowers us to be vigilant and proactive in monitoring medication safety.

Collaboration with healthcare professionals also involves being aware of potential medication-related issues, such as medication non-adherence. By working together, we can develop strategies to overcome barriers to medication adherence, such as memory difficulties, complex medication regimens, or physical limitations. Healthcare professionals can provide guidance on medication reminders, pill organizers, and other tools that can aid in medication management.

Furthermore, healthcare professionals can assist in educating caregivers and family members about medication safety. This education can encompass topics like proper medication storage, potential drug interactions, and recognizing signs of medication-related problems. By arming ourselves with this knowledge, we can play a more active role in safeguarding our loved ones' health.

In conclusion, collaboration with healthcare professionals is crucial for ensuring medication safety in the care of aging loved ones. By working together, we can minimize the risks associated with medication management and enhance the overall well-being of our elderly family members. Let us actively engage with healthcare professionals, seek their guidance, and be proactive advocates for medication safety.

Chapter 9: Fall Prevention and Safety Services for the Elderly

Identifying Fall Risks and Implementing Preventive Measures

Falls are a significant concern for the elderly population, often leading to serious injuries and a decline in overall health and independence. As caregivers, nurses, baby boomers, and grown children, it is crucial to understand the various fall risks faced by the elderly and take proactive measures to prevent these accidents. This subchapter aims to provide you with the knowledge and tools necessary to identify fall risks and implement effective preventive measures for your aging loved ones.

To begin with, it is essential to recognize the common factors that increase the likelihood of falls. These may include physical impairments such as muscle weakness, balance problems, and vision or hearing loss. Additionally, environmental hazards like slippery floors, poor lighting, cluttered pathways, and inadequate bathroom facilities can significantly contribute to falls. By assessing these risk factors, you can create a safer living environment for your elderly loved ones.

Implementing preventive measures starts with home modifications tailored to the specific needs of the individual. Installing grab bars in bathrooms, handrails along stairways, and adequate lighting throughout the house can greatly enhance safety. Removing tripping hazards, such as loose rugs or electrical cords, and securing carpets and mats can also minimize the risk of falls. Furthermore, ensuring that furniture is arranged in a way that allows for easy navigation and access to commonly used items is crucial.

In addition to environmental modifications, promoting physical activity and strength training can improve balance and reduce the risk of falls. Encouraging regular exercise, such as walking or engaging in low-impact activities like tai chi, can help maintain muscle strength and flexibility. Furthermore, regular eye and hearing check-ups can identify any sensory impairments that may contribute to falls.

Medication management plays a vital role in fall prevention as well. Reviewing medications with a healthcare professional can help identify drugs that may cause dizziness or other side effects that increase fall risk. It is important to follow medication schedules strictly and ensure proper storage to avoid any accidental misuse.

Lastly, educating caregivers, family members, and the elderly themselves about fall risks and preventive measures is crucial for comprehensive fall prevention. By raising awareness and providing resources on fall prevention strategies, you empower your loved ones to be proactive in their own safety.

In conclusion, identifying fall risks and implementing preventive measures is essential in ensuring the safety and well-being of the elderly. By understanding the common factors contributing to falls and taking appropriate actions, such as home modifications, promoting physical activity, managing medications, and raising awareness, caregivers, nurses, baby boomers, and grown children can significantly reduce the risk of falls and contribute to a safer and more independent lifestyle for their aging loved ones.

Creating a Safe Environment to Prevent Accidents

Ensuring the safety of our aging loved ones is of utmost importance. As caregivers, nurses, baby boomers, and grown children, it is crucial for us to create a safe environment that minimizes the risk of accidents and promotes the overall well-being of our elderly family members. In this subchapter, we will explore various strategies and tips to help you establish a safe and secure living space for your aging loved ones.

One key aspect of creating a safe environment is to make necessary home modifications. As our loved ones age, their mobility may decrease, making it essential to remove any potential hazards. Installing handrails in hallways and bathrooms, removing clutter, and ensuring proper lighting are simple yet effective ways to prevent accidents such as falls. Additionally, consider arranging furniture in a way that allows for easy navigation and clear pathways throughout the house.

Another vital aspect of safety is medication management. Many elderly individuals require multiple medications, making it crucial to establish a system that ensures they are taking the right dosage at the right time. Create a detailed medication schedule, use pill organizers, and consider utilizing medication management services if needed. Regularly review medications with healthcare professionals to ensure proper usage and minimize the risk of adverse drug interactions.

Meal preparation and nutrition services are equally important in maintaining a safe environment. As our loved ones age, their nutritional needs may change, and they may require assistance with meal planning and preparation. Ensure that meals are well-balanced, healthy, and tailored to any specific dietary requirements. Consider utilizing nutrition services that provide personalized meal plans to ensure your loved ones receive proper nourishment.

Preventing accidents related to dementia or Alzheimer's is a specific concern for many caregivers. Ensure that the living space is secure, with locks on doors and windows to prevent wandering. Install alarms or motion sensors that can alert you if your loved one leaves the house unattended. Labeling cabinets and drawers, using color-coded signs, and creating a daily routine can also help reduce confusion and enhance safety for individuals with cognitive impairments.

Lastly, it is important to educate ourselves and our loved ones about fall prevention and safety measures. Encourage regular exercise to improve strength and balance. Provide assistive devices such as canes or walkers if necessary. Install grab bars in bathrooms and nonslip mats in the shower. Regularly inspect the home for potential hazards and address them promptly.

By implementing these strategies and creating a safe environment, we can significantly reduce the risk of accidents and promote the well-being of our aging loved ones. Remember, a safe home fosters independence, security, and overall happiness for our elderly family members.

Assisting Aging Loved Ones in Maintaining Balance and Mobility

As our loved ones age, it becomes increasingly important to pay attention to their balance and mobility. Falls can have serious consequences, leading to injuries, hospitalizations, and a decline in overall quality of life. As caregivers, nurses, baby boomers, and grown children, it is crucial that we take proactive steps to help our aging loved ones maintain their balance and mobility for as long as possible. In this subchapter, we will discuss various strategies and resources available to assist in this endeavor.

One of the first steps in promoting balance and mobility is to ensure that the home environment is safe and accessible. Simple modifications, such as removing clutter, installing grab bars in bathrooms, and improving lighting, can significantly reduce the risk of falls. Additionally, considering the use of mobility aids, such as canes or walkers, can provide much-needed support and stability.

In-home physical therapy is another valuable resource for maintaining balance and mobility. Physical therapists can develop personalized exercise programs that target specific muscle groups and improve strength, coordination, and flexibility. These exercises can be done in the comfort of the home and can greatly enhance overall physical function.

For those with dementia or Alzheimer's disease, maintaining balance and mobility can be particularly challenging. Caregivers should pay special attention to creating a safe environment, implementing strategies to prevent wandering, and engaging in activities that promote movement and cognitive stimulation. Consulting with specialists in dementia care can provide invaluable guidance and support in managing these unique challenges.

Meal preparation and nutrition services are also essential for maintaining balance and mobility. A well-balanced diet rich in nutrients can help prevent muscle loss and improve overall physical health. Caregivers can seek assistance from nutritionists or meal delivery services to ensure that their loved ones are receiving proper nourishment.

Furthermore, medication management services can play a crucial role in maintaining balance and mobility. Caregivers can consult with healthcare professionals or utilize technology to ensure medications are taken as prescribed, minimizing side effects that may affect mobility.

Lastly, fall prevention and safety services are vital for maintaining balance and mobility. These services can include home assessments, the installation of safety devices, and educational programs to raise awareness about fall risks and prevention strategies. Caregivers should actively seek out these resources to create a safe living environment for their loved ones.

In conclusion, maintaining balance and mobility is of utmost importance for our aging loved ones. By implementing home modifications, engaging in physical therapy, ensuring proper nutrition and medication management, and utilizing fall prevention and safety services, caregivers, nurses, baby boomers, and grown children can make a significant difference in the lives of their aging loved ones. Let us work together to enhance the quality of life for the elderly and ensure their well-being for years to come.

Chapter 10: Emotional Support for Caregivers

Coping with the Emotional Challenges of Caregiving

Introduction:

Being a caregiver for an aging loved one can be a rewarding experience, filled with moments of joy and connection. However, it can also bring about a range of emotional challenges that can take a toll on your well-being. In this subchapter, we will explore some of the common emotional challenges that caregivers face and provide strategies to cope with them effectively.

Understanding the Emotional Challenges:

Caregiving often involves witnessing the decline of a loved one's physical and cognitive abilities, which can be emotionally distressing. Additionally, the demands of caregiving can lead to feelings of overwhelm, guilt, frustration, and even burnout. It is essential to recognize and address these emotions to ensure your own mental health and provide the best care possible.

Strategies for Coping:

1. Seek Support: Reach out to support groups, online forums, or professional counselors who can provide guidance, empathy, and a safe space to share your emotional journey. Surrounding yourself with individuals who understand your challenges can alleviate feelings of isolation.

2. Self-Care: Prioritize self-care by engaging in activities that bring you joy and relaxation. Regular exercise, meditation, hobbies, and quality time with friends and family can help you recharge and manage stress effectively.

3. Set Realistic Expectations: Understand that caregiving is a complex role and accept that you cannot do everything perfectly. Set realistic expectations for yourself and your loved one, and don't hesitate to ask for help when needed.

4. Take Breaks: It's crucial to take regular breaks to prevent burnout. Arrange for respite care or ask family and friends to help out, allowing you to recharge and take care of your own needs.

5. Find Meaning and Purpose: Focus on the positive aspects of caregiving, such as the opportunity to make a difference in your loved one's life. Celebrate small victories and find meaning in the role you play as a caregiver.

Conclusion:

Coping with the emotional challenges of caregiving is a crucial aspect of providing effective care for aging loved ones. By understanding and addressing these challenges, caregivers can ensure their own well-being while continuing to provide compassionate and quality care. Remember, you are not alone on this journey, and seeking support is a sign of strength. Take care of yourself, find balance, and embrace the rewarding moments that caregiving can bring.

Self-Care Strategies for Caregivers

Introduction:

As a caregiver, you play a crucial role in the lives of your aging loved ones. However, it is important to remember that taking care of yourself is just as important as taking care of them. This subchapter will provide you with valuable self-care strategies to ensure that you maintain your physical, emotional, and mental well-being while providing care.

Physical Self-Care:

Caring for an elderly loved one can be physically demanding, so it is essential to prioritize your physical health. Make sure to get regular exercise, eat a balanced diet, and get enough rest. Engage in activities that you enjoy and that help you relax, such as yoga or walking. Remember to take breaks and ask for help when needed, as overexertion can lead to burnout.

Emotional Self-Care:

Being a caregiver can be emotionally draining. It is important to acknowledge and process your emotions. Seek support from friends, family, or support groups who can empathize with your experiences. Take time for yourself to engage in activities that bring you joy and help you recharge. Practice mindfulness and stress-management techniques to help alleviate anxiety and promote emotional well-being.

Mental Self-Care:

Caregiving can be mentally challenging, so it is crucial to prioritize your mental health. Set realistic expectations for yourself and your loved one, and remember that it is okay to ask for help. Engage in activities that stimulate your mind, such as reading or puzzles. Consider seeking professional counseling or therapy to help you navigate the emotional and psychological aspects of caregiving.

Creating Boundaries:

Establishing boundaries is vital for maintaining a healthy caregiver-care recipient relationship. Learn to say no when necessary, and don't feel guilty about taking time for yourself. Delegate tasks to other family members or professionals to alleviate your workload. Communicate openly and honestly with your loved one about your needs and limitations.

Seeking Respite Care:

Respite care offers temporary relief to caregivers by providing professional care for their loved ones. Consider utilizing respite care services to take breaks and rejuvenate. This can be in the form of in-home care, adult day programs, or short-term care facilities. It is essential to take regular breaks to prevent burnout and maintain your overall well-being.

Conclusion:

As a caregiver, you must prioritize your own self-care to ensure that you can provide the best care for your aging loved ones. Remember that you are not alone in this journey, and seeking support is crucial. By implementing these self-care strategies, you can maintain your physical, emotional, and mental health, allowing you to provide the best possible care for your loved ones.

Seeking Support and Resources for Caregiver Well-being

One of the most important aspects of caring for aging loved ones is ensuring that the caregivers themselves receive the support and resources they need to maintain their own well-being. Caregiving can be a physically and emotionally demanding role, and it is crucial for caregivers to prioritize their own health and self-care. This subchapter will explore various support systems and resources available to caregivers, including professional assistance, community programs, and self-care strategies.

For caregivers, seeking support from professionals such as nurses and homecare providers can be immensely beneficial. These professionals can offer guidance, advice, and practical assistance in caring for aging loved ones. Nurses, in particular, are trained to provide specialized care for the elderly and can offer valuable insight into managing conditions such as dementia and Alzheimer's. Additionally, homecare providers can offer in-home physical therapy services to help elderly individuals maintain their mobility and independence.

In addition to professional support, caregivers can also seek assistance from community programs and organizations. Many communities offer services such as home modifications to ensure the safety and accessibility of the elderly, meal preparation and nutrition services, and medication management services. These programs can alleviate some of the caregiver's responsibilities and provide much-needed respite.

Taking care of oneself is essential for caregivers to avoid burnout and maintain their own well-being. This subchapter will also emphasize the importance of self-care strategies for caregivers, such as regular exercise, maintaining a healthy diet, and finding time for relaxation and hobbies. It will provide practical tips and suggestions for incorporating self-care practices into a caregiver's daily routine.

Furthermore, fall prevention and safety services for the elderly will be discussed, as falls are a common concern for aging individuals. This subchapter will provide guidance on creating a safe environment for the elderly, including tips on reducing fall hazards and implementing safety measures.

Overall, this subchapter will serve as a comprehensive guide for caregivers, nurses, baby boomers, and grown children who are involved in homecare for the elderly. It will highlight the importance of seeking support and resources for caregiver well-being, and provide valuable information on various services and programs available to assist caregivers in their role. By prioritizing caregiver well-being, we can ensure that aging loved ones receive the highest quality of care and support they deserve.

Chapter 11: Legal and Financial Considerations

Understanding Legal Documents for Elderly Care

As caregivers, nurses, baby boomers, and grown children, it is vital to have a comprehensive understanding of legal documents related to elderly care. These documents play a crucial role in ensuring the well-being and protection of our aging loved ones. In this subchapter, we will explore the importance of legal documents and their significance in various aspects of homecare for the elderly.

One of the primary legal documents that caregivers should be aware of is the power of attorney. This document grants a designated person the legal authority to make decisions on behalf of the elderly individual when they are no longer able to do so themselves. Understanding the different types of powers of attorney, such as financial and healthcare, is essential for ensuring that the elderly person's wishes are respected and their affairs are managed appropriately.

Another crucial document is the living will or advance healthcare directive. This legal document allows individuals to express their preferences regarding medical treatment and end-of-life care. By understanding and respecting the wishes outlined in the living will, caregivers can ensure that the elderly person's healthcare decisions align with their desires and values.

Additionally, caregivers should familiarize themselves with guardianship and conservatorship. These legal arrangements involve appointing a guardian or conservator to make decisions for individuals who are deemed mentally or physically incapable of managing their own affairs. Understanding the process of obtaining guardianship or conservatorship is vital for offering the necessary care and support to aging loved ones.

Furthermore, this subchapter will delve into the importance of legal documents in relation to specific elderly care niches. For example, dementia care requires caregivers to understand the legal implications of managing a person's finances, ensuring their safety, and making healthcare decisions. In-home physical therapy may require consent forms and waivers to protect both the therapist and the elderly person. Alzheimer's care may involve legal documents pertaining to long-term care facilities and specialized care plans.

Understanding legal documents related to home modifications, meal preparation, medication management, fall prevention, and safety services for the elderly is also crucial. These documents can help caregivers ensure that the necessary modifications are made to the home environment, that proper nutrition and medication management are implemented, and that the elderly person's safety is prioritized.

In conclusion, comprehending legal documents for elderly care is essential for caregivers, nurses, baby boomers, and grown children. These documents provide the necessary legal framework to protect the rights, wishes, and well-being of our aging loved ones. By understanding the significance of power of attorney, living wills, guardianship, and conservatorship, caregivers can navigate the complexities of homecare for the elderly with confidence and ensure the best possible care for their loved ones.

Financial Planning for Aging Loved Ones

As our loved ones age, it becomes increasingly important to plan for their financial well-being. This subchapter will provide valuable guidance on how to effectively manage the financial aspects of caring for aging loved ones. Whether you are a caregiver, nurse, baby boomer, or grown child, understanding the ins and outs of financial planning for the elderly is crucial in providing them with the best care possible.

One of the primary concerns in financial planning for aging loved ones is ensuring they have sufficient funds to cover the costs of their care. This may include expenses such as home modifications, in-home physical therapy, dementia or Alzheimer's care, meal preparation, medication management, and fall prevention and safety services. By carefully assessing their needs and exploring available resources, caregivers can create a comprehensive financial plan that addresses these aspects.

Medicare and Medicaid are essential programs to consider when it comes to financing elderly care. Understanding the eligibility criteria, coverage options, and limitations of these programs is vital to maximize the benefits available to your loved ones. Additionally, exploring long-term care insurance policies can provide financial security and help cover the costs of professional homecare services.

Another crucial aspect of financial planning is ensuring your loved ones have a solid estate plan in place. This includes creating a will, designating a power of attorney, and establishing a healthcare proxy. By discussing these matters with your aging loved ones early on, you can help them make informed decisions about their assets and end-of-life wishes. Seeking legal guidance from an elder law attorney is highly recommended to navigate this complex process.

Planning for the future also involves considering potential healthcare expenses. Exploring options such as health savings accounts (HSAs) or long-term care savings plans can help mitigate the financial burden of medical treatments and services.

Lastly, it is important to regularly review and update the financial plan as circumstances change. Aging loved ones may require additional care or experience changes in their financial situation, so staying proactive and adaptable is key to ensuring their long-term financial stability.

In conclusion, financial planning for aging loved ones is a critical aspect of providing them with the best possible care. By understanding various funding options, maximizing benefits from programs such as Medicare and Medicaid, and creating a comprehensive estate plan, caregivers can effectively manage the financial aspects of caring for the elderly. Regularly reviewing and updating the plan ensures ongoing financial stability as circumstances evolve.

Navigating Long-Term Care Insurance and Government Programs

As caregivers, nurses, baby boomers, and grown children, understanding the complexities of long-term care insurance and government programs is crucial when caring for aging loved ones. This subchapter aims to provide valuable insights into these topics, empowering individuals in the field of homecare for the elderly, dementia care, in-home physical therapy, Alzheimer's care, home modifications, meal preparation, medication management, and fall prevention and safety services.

Long-term care insurance is an essential financial tool that can help cover the costs of care when your loved one requires assistance with daily activities such as bathing, dressing, or eating. This section will explore the key aspects of long-term care insurance, including what it covers, how to select the right policy, and tips for filing claims. We will also discuss the importance of understanding policy limitations, exclusions, and waiting periods to avoid any surprises down the road.

In addition to long-term care insurance, various government programs can provide financial assistance and support to seniors in need. This subchapter will shed light on these programs, including Medicare, Medicaid, and Veterans Affairs benefits. Understanding the eligibility criteria, application process, and benefits of each program will enable caregivers to make informed decisions and access the necessary resources to ensure quality care for their loved ones.

Furthermore, this subchapter will address common challenges and pitfalls caregivers may encounter when dealing with long-term care insurance and government programs. From handling claim denials to navigating complex paperwork, we will provide practical tips and strategies to overcome these hurdles. Additionally, we will discuss the importance of staying updated with changing policies and regulations, as these can significantly impact the availability and coverage of services.

Lastly, we will explore resources and organizations that caregivers can turn to for assistance and guidance. These include local agencies on aging, non-profit organizations, and online support groups. By tapping into these resources, caregivers can access expert advice, connect with others facing similar challenges, and find the help they need to ensure their aging loved ones receive the best possible care.

In conclusion, understanding the intricacies of long-term care insurance and government programs is vital for caregivers, nurses, baby boomers, and grown children involved in homecare for the elderly. This subchapter aims to equip readers with the knowledge and tools they need to navigate these systems effectively, ensuring that their loved ones receive the necessary care while alleviating financial burdens.

Chapter 12: Future Planning and Transitions

Preparing for Transitions in Care

As caregivers, nurses, baby boomers, and grown children, we understand the importance of providing the best possible care for our aging loved ones. One crucial aspect of this responsibility is preparing for transitions in care. Whether it's moving our loved ones to a nursing home, transitioning from hospital to home, or simply adjusting to new healthcare needs, careful planning and preparation can make these transitions smoother and less stressful for both the elderly and their caregivers.

When it comes to homecare for the elderly, transitions may occur due to various reasons such as declining health, the need for specialized care, or changes in living arrangements. It's essential to anticipate and plan for these transitions in advance, ensuring that the necessary support and resources are readily available. This includes researching and identifying reputable homecare agencies or facilities that align with your loved one's needs and preferences. Engaging in open and honest communication with your loved one about their desires and wishes will also help in making informed decisions during such transitions.

For those caring for elderly individuals with dementia or Alzheimer's, transitions in care can be particularly challenging. Consistency and familiarity are key in providing comfort and reducing anxiety for these individuals. Establishing routines, maintaining familiar surroundings, and ensuring continuity of care are vital during transitions. Seeking support from dementia care specialists and joining support groups can also provide valuable guidance and assistance throughout the process.

In-home physical therapy is often a crucial component of elderly care, especially following an injury or surgery. When transitioning from a hospital or rehabilitation center to home, it's essential to have a plan in place to seamlessly continue physical therapy at home. This may involve coordinating with healthcare professionals, ensuring the availability of necessary equipment, and creating a safe and conducive environment for therapy sessions.

Transitions in care also necessitate a focus on nutrition, medication management, fall prevention, and overall safety for the elderly. Meal preparation and nutrition services can help ensure that your loved one receives a well-balanced and nourishing diet, supporting their overall health and well-being. Medication management services can assist in organizing and administering medications correctly, reducing the risk of medication errors. Implementing fall prevention strategies and making necessary home modifications, such as installing handrails or removing trip hazards, can significantly enhance safety and prevent accidents.

In conclusion, preparing for transitions in care requires careful planning, open communication, and a focus on meeting the specific needs of our aging loved ones. Whether it's arranging homecare, managing transitions in dementia care, continuing physical therapy at home, or ensuring proper nutrition and medication management, being proactive in anticipating and addressing these transitions will contribute to a smoother and more comfortable caregiving journey for both caregivers and their elderly loved ones.

End-of-Life Planning and Hospice Care

As caregivers, nurses, baby boomers, and grown children, we often find ourselves faced with the difficult task of planning for the end-of-life care of our aging loved ones. It is an emotionally challenging and sensitive topic, but one that must be addressed to ensure the comfort and dignity of our loved ones during their final days. This subchapter aims to provide guidance and information on end-of-life planning and the invaluable role of hospice care.

End-of-life planning involves making decisions about medical treatments, financial matters, and personal preferences for care. It is crucial to have open and honest conversations with our loved ones about their wishes, including their preferences for medical interventions, life-sustaining treatments, and funeral arrangements. This planning process helps alleviate the burden on family members and ensures that the individual's desires are respected.

Hospice care is an approach to end-of-life care that focuses on providing comfort and support to individuals with a terminal illness. This compassionate care is delivered by a team of professionals, including doctors, nurses, social workers, and spiritual advisors. Hospice care can be provided either at home or in a specialized facility, catering to the unique needs and preferences of the individual.

For caregivers, understanding the benefits and services offered by hospice care is crucial. Hospice care provides pain and symptom management, emotional support for both the individual and their family, assistance with daily activities, and spiritual guidance. The goal of hospice care is to improve the quality of life for individuals facing a terminal illness and to offer support to their families during this challenging time.

In addition to hospice care, it is essential to consider other supportive services that can enhance the end-of-life experience for our loved ones. These may include in-home physical therapy to maintain mobility and comfort, home modifications to ensure a safe and accessible environment, meal preparation and nutrition services to meet dietary needs, medication management to ensure proper dosing and administration, and fall prevention and safety services to minimize the risk of accidents.

As caregivers, nurses, baby boomers, and grown children, we have a responsibility to prioritize the well-being and comfort of our aging loved ones. By understanding the importance of end-of-life planning and the benefits of hospice care, we can provide the support and guidance necessary to ensure a peaceful and dignified journey for our loved ones in their final days.

Resources for Grief Support and Bereavement

Caring for an aging loved one can be emotionally challenging, especially when faced with the inevitable loss of a loved one. Grief and bereavement are natural responses to loss, and it is important for caregivers, nurses, baby boomers, and grown children to have access to resources that can provide support during this difficult time. This subchapter aims to provide an overview of various resources available to individuals involved in homecare for the elderly, dementia care, in-home physical therapy, Alzheimer's care, home modifications, meal preparation and nutrition services, medication management, and fall prevention and safety services.

One valuable resource for grief support and bereavement is local hospice agencies. These organizations specialize in end-of-life care and can offer counseling and support to both caregivers and their loved ones. Hospice agencies often provide bereavement support groups, individual counseling, and educational materials to help individuals navigate the grieving process.

Another helpful resource is online grief support communities and forums. These platforms allow caregivers and others to connect with individuals who are experiencing or have experienced similar losses. Online communities provide a safe space to share stories, seek advice, and find comfort in the company of others who understand their grief.

Various national organizations, such as the American Association of Retired Persons (AARP) and the Alzheimer's Association, offer resources specifically tailored to support caregivers and families dealing with dementia, Alzheimer's disease, and other memory-related illnesses. These organizations provide information, educational materials, support hotlines, and local support groups to help caregivers cope with the challenges of caring for someone with dementia.

Additionally, many local communities have grief support centers or counseling services that offer individual or group counseling sessions for those experiencing grief. These centers often have licensed therapists or counselors who specialize in grief and bereavement and can provide valuable support and guidance.

Lastly, it is important to mention the availability of professional grief counselors and therapists who specialize in grief and bereavement. These professionals can offer individualized support and counseling tailored to the unique needs of each caregiver or family member.

In conclusion, when facing the loss of a loved one, it is crucial for caregivers, nurses, baby boomers, and grown children to have access to grief support and bereavement resources. From local hospice agencies and online communities to national organizations and professional counselors, there are numerous resources available to provide the support and guidance needed during this difficult time. By utilizing these resources, caregivers and family members can find solace, understanding, and the tools necessary to navigate their grief journey.

Chapter 13: Additional Resources and Support

Local Community Resources for Elderly Care

As caregivers, nurses, baby boomers, and grown children, it is crucial to be aware of the local community resources available to provide the best care for our aging loved ones. These resources can greatly assist in ensuring their overall well-being, safety, and quality of life. This subchapter aims to highlight some valuable local community resources that cater to various needs of elderly individuals, including homecare, dementia care, physical therapy, Alzheimer's care, home modifications, nutrition services, medication management, and fall prevention.

When it comes to homecare for the elderly, several local organizations and agencies provide services such as personal care, companionship, and assistance with daily activities. These services can help seniors maintain their independence and age comfortably in their own homes. Additionally, there are specialized programs and facilities that focus on dementia care, offering support and specialized care for individuals with cognitive impairments.

In-home physical therapy is another essential resource for the elderly. Many local physical therapy clinics offer home visits, enabling seniors to receive professional rehabilitation services without leaving the comfort of their homes. This can be highly beneficial for those with mobility issues or chronic conditions.

For individuals diagnosed with Alzheimer's, local community resources often include support groups, memory care centers, and respite care services. These resources not only provide relief to the primary caregivers but also offer specialized care and activities for individuals with Alzheimer's, enhancing their cognitive abilities and overall quality of life.

Home modifications are vital for creating a safe and comfortable environment for the elderly. Local organizations provide assistance in modifying homes to be more accessible, such as installing grab bars, ramps, and stairlifts, to prevent accidents and improve mobility.

Proper nutrition is crucial for the overall health and well-being of the elderly. Local meal preparation and nutrition services deliver nutritious meals to seniors' homes, ensuring they receive a balanced diet and meet their dietary requirements.

Medication management services help seniors organize and take their medications correctly, minimizing the risk of medication errors and adverse effects. These services can include medication reminders, delivery, and consultations with pharmacists.

Lastly, fall prevention and safety services are essential to minimize the risk of falls, which are a leading cause of injury among the elderly. Local organizations provide home safety assessments, offer suggestions for modifications, and educate seniors on fall prevention techniques.

By being aware of these local community resources, caregivers, nurses, baby boomers, and grown children can ensure that their aging loved ones receive the best possible care. These resources not only address specific needs but also provide support, education, and peace of mind for both the seniors and their caregivers.

Support Groups and Online Communities

Caregiving for aging loved ones can be a challenging and emotional journey. It is a role that often comes with immense responsibilities, complex decisions, and feelings of isolation. However, you are not alone in this journey. Support groups and online communities can provide a valuable network of understanding individuals who can offer guidance, advice, and emotional support.

Support groups are a vital resource for caregivers, nurses, baby boomers, and grown children alike. These groups bring together individuals who are facing similar challenges and provide a safe space to share experiences, frustrations, and triumphs. They offer a sense of belonging and understanding that can be difficult to find elsewhere. By participating in support groups, caregivers can gain valuable insight into effective caregiving techniques, learn about available resources, and find comfort in knowing that others are going through similar experiences.

Online communities have become increasingly popular in recent years, offering a convenient option for individuals to connect and engage with others facing similar caregiving situations. These communities provide a platform for open discussions, where caregivers can seek advice, ask questions, and share their own experiences. Online communities also offer the advantage of anonymity, allowing individuals to freely express their thoughts and concerns without fear of judgment.

For caregivers in the niche of homecare for the elderly, online communities and support groups can be particularly beneficial. These platforms allow caregivers to exchange information and learn about best practices in providing in-home physical therapy, dementia care, Alzheimer's care, and fall prevention and safety services. Caregivers can also gain insights into home modifications that can enhance the safety and accessibility of their loved ones' living environment.

Moreover, support groups and online communities can also be a valuable resource for caregivers seeking guidance on meal preparation and nutrition services for the elderly, as well as medication management services. By connecting with other caregivers, nurses, and professionals in these areas, caregivers can access a wealth of knowledge and practical advice.

In conclusion, support groups and online communities are essential for caregivers, nurses, baby boomers, and grown children involved in homecare for the elderly. These platforms provide a supportive network, invaluable information, and emotional support for those facing the challenges of caregiving. By joining these communities, caregivers can find solace, gain insight, and connect with others who truly understand their journey.

Professional Services for Elderly Caregivers

As a caregiver for an aging loved one, you may find yourself overwhelmed with the responsibilities and challenges that come with providing care. However, there are professional services available that can offer support and assistance to both you and your elderly loved one. This subchapter aims to introduce various professional services for elderly caregivers that can greatly enhance the quality of care and overall well-being of your loved one.

One crucial professional service for elderly caregivers is homecare for the elderly. Homecare services provide trained and experienced caregivers who can assist with daily activities such as bathing, dressing, meal preparation, and medication management. These professionals not only ensure the safety and comfort of your loved one but also provide companionship and emotional support.

For those dealing with dementia or Alzheimer's, specialized care is essential. Dementia care services offer tailored support to individuals with memory loss, focusing on cognitive stimulation, behavior management, and maintaining a safe environment. These professionals possess the skills and knowledge necessary to handle the unique challenges associated with these conditions.

In-home physical therapy services are another valuable resource for elderly caregivers. Physical therapists can design personalized exercise programs to improve mobility, strength, and balance. They can also address specific issues like pain management and fall prevention, helping your loved one maintain their independence and overall well-being.

Home modifications for the elderly are crucial to ensure a safe and accessible living environment. Professional services can assess your loved one's home and recommend modifications such as installing grab bars, ramps, and non-slip flooring. These modifications minimize the risk of accidents and make daily activities easier for your loved one.

Meal preparation and nutrition services are also vital for the elderly. Nutritional experts can create balanced meal plans tailored to your loved one's dietary needs, ensuring they receive proper nutrition. These services can also include grocery shopping and meal delivery, relieving you of the burden of meal preparation.

Medication management services help elderly caregivers ensure their loved ones take the correct medications at the right times. Professionals can organize medication schedules, provide reminders, and monitor for any adverse effects or potential interactions.

Lastly, fall prevention and safety services play a crucial role in keeping your loved one safe. These professionals can conduct home safety assessments, identify potential hazards, and recommend strategies to minimize the risk of falls. They may also provide education on fall prevention techniques and offer assistive devices like walkers or canes.

In conclusion, professional services for elderly caregivers are invaluable resources that can significantly enhance the care provided to aging loved ones. Whether you require assistance with homecare, specialized dementia care, physical therapy, home modifications, meal preparation, medication management, or fall prevention, these services offer a range of support tailored to your specific needs. By utilizing these professional services, you can ensure the well-being, safety, and comfort of your loved one while alleviating some of the burdens associated with caregiving.

Chapter 14: Conclusion

Recap of Key Points

In this subchapter, we will summarize the key points discussed throughout the book "Caring for Aging Loved Ones: A Guide to Homecare for the Elderly." This recap aims to provide caregivers, nurses, baby boomers, and grown children with a quick overview of the essential information covered in the book.

1. Understanding Homecare for the Elderly:
- The importance of personalized care in the comfort of one's own home.
- Benefits of homecare, including maintaining independence and promoting emotional well-being.

2. Dementia Care for the Elderly:

- Recognizing the signs and symptoms of dementia.

- Strategies for effective communication and managing challenging behaviors.

- Creating a safe and stimulating environment for individuals with dementia.

3. In-Home Physical Therapy for the Elderly:

- The role of physical therapy in improving mobility, balance, and strength.

- Exercises and techniques for promoting independence and preventing falls.

- Collaborating with healthcare professionals to develop personalized therapy plans.

4. Alzheimer's Care for the Elderly:

- Understanding the stages and progression of Alzheimer's disease.

- Techniques for managing memory loss, confusion, and agitation.

- Providing emotional support to both the individual with Alzheimer's and their family.

5. Home Modifications for the Elderly:

- Adapting the home environment to promote safety and accessibility.

- Installing grab bars, ramps, and other assistive devices.

- Creating a barrier-free space for seniors with mobility challenges.

6. Meal Preparation and Nutrition Services for the Elderly:

- The importance of a balanced and nutritious diet for seniors.

- Tips for meal planning, grocery shopping, and cooking for older adults.

- Utilizing meal delivery services or hiring a personal chef to ensure adequate nutrition.

7. Medication Management Services for the Elderly:

- The significance of medication adherence and avoiding potential drug interactions.

- Organizing medication schedules and utilizing pill organizers.

- Working with healthcare professionals to ensure proper medication management.

8. Fall Prevention and Safety Services for the Elderly:

- Identifying common fall hazards in the home and implementing preventive measures.

- Encouraging regular exercise and balance training.

- Engaging in regular home safety assessments and modifications.

By reviewing these key points, caregivers, nurses, baby boomers, and grown children can gain a comprehensive understanding of the various aspects of homecare for the elderly. Implementing the knowledge gained from this book will empower them to provide the best possible care and support for their aging loved ones, ensuring their safety, well-being, and quality of life.

Encouragement and Support for Caregivers

Introduction:

Being a caregiver for an aging loved one can be both rewarding and challenging. It requires immense dedication, patience, and selflessness, as well as a deep understanding of the needs and struggles of the elderly. In this subchapter, we will explore various ways to provide encouragement and support to caregivers, ensuring they can stay motivated and resilient in their caregiving journey.

1. Recognizing the Importance of Self-Care:

Caregivers often prioritize the needs of their loved ones above their own, often neglecting their physical, emotional, and mental well-being. It is crucial to emphasize the significance of self-care and encourage caregivers to take breaks, seek respite care, and engage in activities that bring them joy and relaxation. By prioritizing self-care, caregivers can maintain their own health and well-being, enabling them to provide better care to their aging loved ones.

2. Building a Support Network:

Caregivers often feel isolated and overwhelmed with their responsibilities. By connecting with other caregivers, nurses, and professionals in the field, they can share experiences, seek advice, and find empathy. Support groups, online forums, and caregiver networks can provide a platform for caregivers to connect and share their challenges and triumphs, creating a sense of belonging and understanding.

3. Education and Training:

Providing caregivers with access to educational resources and training programs can empower them with knowledge and skills to better support their aging loved ones. Workshops and seminars on topics such as dementia care, in-home physical therapy, Alzheimer's care, and fall prevention can equip caregivers with practical techniques and strategies, boosting their confidence and enhancing the quality of care they provide.

4. Respite Care and Professional Assistance:

Encouraging caregivers to seek respite care services can offer much-needed relief and rejuvenation. Respite care providers can step in temporarily, allowing caregivers to take breaks, attend appointments, or simply have time for themselves. Additionally, professional assistance such as home modifications, meal preparation, medication management, and safety services can alleviate the burden on caregivers, ensuring their loved ones receive the best care possible.

Conclusion:

Caregivers play a vital role in the lives of aging loved ones, often sacrificing their own well-being in the process. By providing encouragement and support, we can help caregivers navigate the challenges they face, ensuring they feel valued, empowered, and equipped to provide the best care possible. Remember, caring for the caregiver ultimately leads to better care for the elderly, fostering a nurturing and loving environment for everyone involved.

Final Thoughts on Caring for Aging Loved Ones

As caregivers, nurses, baby boomers, and grown children, we have embarked on a journey of love and compassion in caring for our aging loved ones. Throughout this book, "Caring for Aging Loved Ones: A Guide to Homecare for the Elderly," we have explored various aspects of homecare, dementia care, physical therapy, Alzheimer's care, home modifications, meal preparation, medication management, fall prevention, and safety services for the elderly. Now, as we reach the end of this guide, let us reflect on our journey and share some final thoughts.

Caring for aging loved ones is not an easy task. It requires patience, understanding, and sacrifice. It can be physically and emotionally draining, but it is also immensely rewarding. The love and care we provide to our elderly family members contribute to their quality of life and well-being. Remember, our role as caregivers is not only to meet their physical needs but also to provide emotional support and companionship.

One of the key lessons we have learned is the importance of education and professional help. By acquiring knowledge about the specific needs and challenges faced by our aging loved ones, we can better tailor our caregiving approach. Seeking advice from healthcare professionals, attending support groups, and utilizing specialized services such as in-home physical therapy, dementia care, or Alzheimer's care can significantly improve the quality of care we provide.

Another crucial aspect we must consider is safety and home modifications. Aging loved ones are more susceptible to falls and accidents, so it is essential to create a safe environment within their homes. Home modifications such as grab bars, non-slip flooring, and adequate lighting can greatly reduce the risk of falls and enhance their independence.

Nutrition and medication management are also vital components of caregiving. Ensuring that our loved ones receive balanced meals and proper nutrition can positively impact their overall health. Additionally, managing medications accurately, organizing pillboxes, and keeping track of doctor appointments are crucial to avoid any potential complications.

Finally, we must not overlook the importance of self-care as caregivers. It is essential to take breaks, seek respite care, and prioritize our own physical and emotional well-being. By caring for ourselves, we can continue providing the best care for our aging loved ones.

In conclusion, caring for aging loved ones is a noble and challenging task. Through this guide, we have explored various aspects of homecare, dementia care, physical therapy, Alzheimer's care, home modifications, meal preparation, medication management, fall prevention, and safety services. By staying informed, seeking professional help, ensuring safety, and practicing self-care, we can make this journey a fulfilling and meaningful one for both our loved ones and ourselves.

Because We Care!
D.W. Lindsey

All rights reserved
First Edition, 2023
© D.W. Lindsey, 2023

No part of this publication may be reproduced, or stored in
a retrieval system, or transmitted in any form by means of
electronic, mechanical, photocopying or otherwise, without
prior written permission from the author.